COMPLETE GUIDE TO UNDERSTANDING DENTAL IMPLANT SURGERY

Comprehensive Insights Into Expert Techniques, Aftercare Tips, Recovery Guidance For Successful Outcomes And Optimal Oral Health

KLEIN HOYLE

© [KLEIN HOYLE] [2024]

All rights reserved.

No part of this book may be reproduced, distributed, or transmitted in any form or by any means, including photocopying, recording, or other electronic or mechanical methods, without the publisher's prior written permission, with the exception of brief quotations in critical reviews and certain other noncommercial uses permitted by copyright law.

Disclaimer

The content in this book is based on the author's expertise and comprehension of the topic. The author has no affiliation or link with any corporation, business, or person. This book is meant to give general information and educational material only, and it should not be interpreted as professional medical advice. Always seek the advice of a skilled healthcare expert if you have any queries about medical issues or treatments. The author and publisher expressly disclaim any responsibility resulting directly or indirectly from the use or use of the information included in this book.

Table of Contents

CHAPTER 1 15
Introduction To Dental Implant Surgery 15
Understanding The Fundamentals Of Dental Implants 15
Historical Background And Development.........17
Benefits And Advantages Of Dental Implants....19
Common Misconceptions And Myths..............22

CHAPTER 2 27
Anatomy Of The Oral Cavity 27
Overview Of Oral Anatomy Relevant For Dental Implants 27
Dental, Gum, And Jawbone Structures............27
The Importance Of Bone Density And Quality ..29
How Dental Anatomy Affects Implant Placement 30

CHAPTER 3 33
Assessment And Planning For Implants 33
Initial Consultation And Assessment 33
Diagnostic Tools Include X-Rays And CT Scans 34
Factors Influencing Treatment Planning 36

A Collaborative Approach Between Dentists And Surgeons 37

CHAPTER 4 39

Types Of Dental Implants 39

Difference Between Endosteal And Subperiosteal Implants 39

Materials For Implant Construction 41

Implant Shapes And Sizes 42

Choosing The Correct Type Of Implant For Specific Cases 43

CHAPTER 5 47

Preparing For Surgery 47

Preoperative Instructions And Guidelines 47

Importance Of Oral Hygiene Before Surgery 48

Potential Lifestyle Adjustments 49

Anesthesia Options And Their Implications 50

CHAPTER 6 53

Surgical Procedure 53

Step-By-Step Explanation Of Implant Implantation 53

   1. Initial Examination and Assessment: 53

   3. Anesthesia: 54

4. Incision: 54
6. Implant Placement: 54
7. Closing the Incision: 55
8. Healing phase: 55
9. Final Restoration: 55
Surgical Techniques 55
   Flapless surgery 55
   Guided Surgery 56
Bone Grafting, Sinus Augmentation 56
Suturing And Closing The Surgical Site 57
   Suturing Techniques: 58
   Post-operative Care: 58
CHAPTER 7 59
Postoperative Care And Recovery 59
Immediate Post-Operative Instructions 59
   1. Bleeding: 59
   2. Pain Management: 60
   3. Swelling: 60
   4. Rest and Recovery: 60
   5. Oral Hygiene: 60
   6. Dietary Restrictions: 61

7. Avoid Smoking and drinking: 61
Managing Pain And Discomfort 61
   1. Take Pain Medication: 62
   2. Apply Ice Packs: 62
   3. Use Over-the-counter Pain Relievers: 62
   4. Rest: 62
   5. Follow Post-Operative Instructions: 63
Diet Recommendations During The Healing Phase
.... 63
   1. Stick to Soft Foods: 63
   2. Avoid Hard or Crunchy Foods: 64
   4. Limit Sugar Consumption: 64
   5. Follow Your Dentist's Recommendations: .. 64
Follow-Up Appointments And Tracking Progress
.... 65
   1. Post-Operative Evaluation: 65
   2. X-rays: 65
   3. Adjustments: 66
   4. Long-Term Care Planning: 66
   5. Addressing Concerns: 66
CHAPTER 8 67

Potential Complications And How To Manage Them 67

Common Complications 67

Early Signs Of Complications And When To Seek Help 68

    1. Prolonged Pain: 68

    2. Swelling: 69

    3. Bleeding: 69

    4. Difficulty Chewing or Speaking: 69

    5. Loose Implant: 69

Strategies To Minimize Risks During And After Surgery 70

    1. Choose a Qualified Provider: 70

    2. Follow Pre- and Post-Operative recommendations: 70

    3. Maintain Good Oral Hygiene: 70

    4. Avoid Smoking and Alcohol: 70

    5. Attend Follow-Up visits: 71

Long-Term Management Of Complications 71

CHAPTER 9 73

Dental Implant Maintenance And Long-Term Care 73

Importance Of Dental Hygiene For Implant Longevity 73
Regular Check-Ups And Professional Cleaning .75
Addressing Issues Such As Peri-Implantitis.......76
Tips To Protect Implants From Damage...........78
    1. Avoid chewing on hard items: 78
    2. Wear a mouthguard: 78
    3. Quit smoking: 79

CHAPTER 10 81
Future Advancements In Dental Implant Technology 81
Current Trends And Research In Implant Dentistry 81
Predicted Advancements In Materials And Techniques 83
The Potential Impact Of Technology................85
Implications For Patient Care And Treatment Outcomes..86
Conclusion 89

THE END 92

ABOUT THIS BOOK

The "Complete Guide to Understanding Dental Implant Surgery" is a must-read for everyone interested in contemporary dentistry, shedding light on the complexities of a transformational surgery that combines science, creativity, and patient care. This comprehensive study, divided into 10 beautifully produced parts, takes readers on a trip from the origins of dental implants to future visions, serving as a useful resource for both dental professionals and patients.

Chapter 1 begins this journey with an intellectual investigation of the fundamental principles, including the history, advantages, and prevalent misunderstandings about dental implants. By digging into the annals of dental history, readers get a comprehensive understanding of how this groundbreaking technology has grown, creating a solid foundation for the next chapters.

As the story progresses, Chapter 2 digs into the complex terrain of oral anatomy, revealing a tapestry of structures critical to the success of dental implant surgery. Through a sophisticated examination of tooth, gum, and jawbone architecture, readers get a thorough grasp of how the interaction of these factors influences implant placement and long-term viability.

Transitioning fluidly, Chapter 3 serves as a light of direction in the maze of evaluation and planning, emphasizing the significance of rigorous assessment and collaborative synergy among dental professionals. Readers will explore diagnostic tools, treatment planning intricacies, and the symbiotic interaction between dentist and surgeon, establishing the groundwork for educated decision-making.

Chapter 4, with its scientific discussion of the many kinds of dental implants, serves as a compass for navigating the complex terrain of implantology. From the distinction between endosteal and subperiosteal implants to the complexities of material selection and implant shape, readers will be equipped to traverse the maze of implant possibilities with confidence and discernment.

With preparations beginning, Chapter 5 emerges as a beacon of readiness, providing patients and practitioners alike with the information they need to traverse the pre-operative terrain with confidence and effectiveness. Readers are well-prepared for the surgical adventure ahead thanks to a thoughtful combination of pre-operative instructions, lifestyle changes, and anesthetic alternatives.

Beginning with the surgical journey in Chapter 6, readers are led through a careful choreography of implant placement, with each step filled with precision and purpose. This chapter acts as a compass, leading practitioners through the varied landscape of surgical intervention, covering everything from surgical methods to bone grafting intricacies.

Navigating the post-operative terrain, Chapter 7 emerges as a beacon of care and recovery, providing comfort and direction in the aftermath of surgical attempts. With insights into immediate post-operative care, pain management measures, and nutritional concerns, readers are guided through the delicate dance of recovery with grace and certainty.

As the trip progresses, Chapter 8 emerges as a beacon of caution, exposing the many traps and hazards that may arise on the road to implantology. Through an honest examination of difficulties and mitigation measures, readers are enabled to face hardship with perseverance and commitment, assuring the length and success of their implant initiatives.

Chapter 9 easily transitions into the world of long-term care, demonstrating that prevention is indeed the best treatment. Readers are given the means to protect their implants from the ravages of time thanks to a mix of insights on implant management, frequent check-ups, and preventative treatments against peri-implantitis.

As the adventure concludes, Chapter 10 looks forward, providing intriguing insights into the future of implantology. From the perspective of cutting-edge research to the revolutionary potential of future technologies, readers are welcomed on a journey of discovery in which the bounds of possibility are constantly redefined.

In conclusion, the "Complete Guide to Understanding Dental Implant Surgery" goes beyond the scope of a textbook, emerging as a beacon of enlightenment and empowerment in the ever-changing world of implant dentistry. This magnum work, with its scientific discourse, practical insights, and visionary view, exemplifies knowledge's transformational potential in molding the future of dental care.

CHAPTER 1

Introduction To Dental Implant Surgery

Understanding The Fundamentals Of Dental Implants

Dental implants are ground-breaking options for restoring lost teeth. But, what precisely are they? Dental implants are titanium posts that are surgically implanted into the jawbone under the gums. These posts serve as prosthetic tooth roots, providing a solid basis for replacement teeth like crowns or dentures.

The procedure of receiving dental implants usually entails many phases. First, your dentist will evaluate your dental health and decide if you are a good candidate for implants. This might include X-rays and scans to assess the health of your jawbone and surrounding tissues.

Once it has been decided that you are a suitable candidate, the implant will be surgically placed. This entails creating an incision in the gum tissue to expose the jawbone, drilling a hole for the implant, and firmly inserting it into the bone. After the implant is put, the gum tissue is sewn back in place, and the healing process starts.

During the healing phase, which might span many months, the implant merges with the surrounding bone, a process known as osseointegration. This is critical for the stability and lifespan of the implant. After the implant has completely integrated with the bone, the final restoration (such as a crown or denture) is connected to the implant to complete the procedure.

One of the primary benefits of dental implants is that they seem, feel, and operate exactly like natural teeth. Unlike conventional dentures or bridges, implants are permanently secured in the jawbone, so they will not slide or move during eating or speaking. This gives patients more comfort and confidence in their smiles.

Furthermore, dental implants promote bone health by stimulating the jawbone, avoiding bone loss that occurs when teeth are absent. This helps to retain the natural structure of the face and avoids the sunken look that may come with standard tooth replacement techniques.

It's essential to realize that, although dental implants have many advantages, they may not be right for everyone. Overall health, dental hygiene practices, and jawbone quality all have an impact on whether implants are a suitable choice for you. A consultation with a knowledgeable dentist or oral surgeon is the best method to decide if dental implants are the best option for repairing your smile.

Historical Background And Development

The notion of dental implants isn't new. There is evidence of early efforts at tooth replacement dating back thousands of years. Archaeological discoveries have shown that ancient civilizations such as the

Mayans and Egyptians employed a variety of materials, including shells and ivory, to make primitive implants.

However, it wasn't until the twentieth century that considerable advances in dental implant technology occurred. In the 1950s, Per-Ingvar Brånemark, a Swedish orthopedic surgeon, produced a significant discovery that revolutionized the area of implant dentistry. Brånemark's studies on bone tissue healing revealed titanium's unique ability to merge with bone, a process he named osseointegration.

This finding established the basis for current dental implantology. Brånemark's pioneering work resulted in the first commercially successful dental implant system, the Brånemark System, debuted in the 1980s. Since then, dental implant technology has evolved and improved, with new materials, procedures, and implant designs always emerging.

Today, dental implants are regarded as the gold standard for tooth replacement, with success rates reaching 95% in most situations. Advances in imaging technologies, such as cone beam computed tomography (CBCT), have made implant design and placement more accurate and predictable than before. Furthermore, advances in implant surface coatings and design have improved osseointegration and reduced healing durations.

The area of implant dentistry is always evolving, with new research aiming at enhancing implant materials, procedures, and results. With continuing innovation and breakthroughs, dental implants are expected to remain the favored choice for repairing smiles for many years.

Benefits And Advantages Of Dental Implants

Dental implants provide several advantages to people who are missing one or more teeth. One of the key benefits of implants is their ability to replicate the look and function of natural teeth. Unlike conventional dentures or bridges, which rest on top of the gums and may be bulky or painful, implants are firmly attached to the jawbone, giving a strong foundation for replacement teeth.

This stability enables patients to eat, talk, and smile confidently, without fear of their teeth sliding or changing out of position. Furthermore, since implants are incorporated into the jawbone, they contribute to bone health and prevent bone loss that may occur when teeth are absent. This helps to retain the natural structure of the face and avoids the sunken look that may come with standard tooth replacement techniques.

Another benefit of dental implants is their durability. Dental implants, with appropriate care and maintenance, may last a lifetime, making them an affordable long-term alternative. Unlike dentures or bridges, which may need to be renewed every 5-10 years, implants are built to endure the rigors of everyday usage and may offer permanent tooth replacement for qualified applicants.

Furthermore, dental implants are very adaptable, able to replace a single tooth, numerous teeth, or even a complete arch of teeth. This makes them appropriate for a broad spectrum of individuals with varied levels of tooth loss. Whether you are missing one or more teeth, implants may be tailored to your specific requirements and restore your smile to its full potential.

Dental implants provide outstanding cosmetic effects. Implants fit easily with your existing teeth, giving a gorgeous, natural-looking smile. Whether you're engaging with friends, family, or coworkers, you can be certain that your smile looks and feels just as it did before you lost your teeth.

In addition to their practical advantages, dental implants provide considerable oral health benefits. Unlike conventional tooth replacement treatments such as bridges, implants do not need the modification or removal of neighboring teeth. This helps to protect the integrity of your natural teeth and reduces the likelihood of issues in the future.

Overall, dental implants provide full treatment for missing teeth, with various advantages to both oral health and quality of life. Whether you need to replace a single tooth or repair your whole smile, implants can help you have the attractive, functional smile you deserve.

Common Misconceptions And Myths

Despite their various advantages, dental implants are sometimes associated with misunderstandings and falsehoods. Understanding the facts behind these myths is critical for making sound choices regarding your dental health. Let us dispel some of the most frequent fallacies regarding dental implants.

Myth No. 1: Dental implants are uncomfortable. While dental implant surgery can cause some discomfort, most patients experience little pain throughout the process. Your dentist will use a local anesthetic to numb the region, assuring your comfort during the procedure. Furthermore, improvements in anesthetic and sedative procedures have made the implant installation procedure more pleasant than ever before.

Myth #2: Dental implants are costly. While dental implants may be more expensive in the beginning than other tooth replacement choices, such as dentures or bridges, they are often more cost-effective over time. This is because implants are intended to last a lifetime with good care, but alternative solutions may need replacement every 5-10 years. Furthermore, many dental insurance policies now cover a percentage of the cost of dental implants, making them more accessible to qualifying patients.

Myth #3: Dental implants have a long healing time. While dental implant surgery does need some healing and osseointegration, most patients may return to regular activities within a few days to a week following the treatment. Your dentist will provide you with post-operative guidelines to help you feel less pain and recuperate faster. With careful care and maintenance, your implants should completely integrate with the bone within a few months, allowing you to enjoy the advantages of a restored smile.

Myth #4: Dental implants are unsuitable for elderly persons. Age is not always a barrier to receiving dental implants. Regardless of your age, if you have excellent general health and enough jawbone density, you may be a candidate for implants. Many older persons find that dental implants increase their quality of life by allowing them to eat, talk, and smile confidently.

Myth #5: Dental implants are high-maintenance. Contrary to common assumptions, dental implants need very little upkeep. Implants may last a lifetime if they are cared for properly, such as brushing, flossing, and seeing the dentist regularly. There is no need for specific cleaning solutions or adhesives, such as those used with dentures. Simply care for your implants as you would your natural teeth, and they will continue to provide you with a beautiful, functioning smile for years to come.

By removing these myths and misunderstandings, you can make an educated decision regarding whether dental implants are the best option for repairing your smile. Consulting with a trained dentist or oral surgeon is the best approach to learning more about your choices and choosing the best treatment plan for your specific circumstances.

CHAPTER 2

Anatomy Of The Oral Cavity

Overview Of Oral Anatomy Relevant For Dental Implants

Understanding the anatomy of the mouth cavity is critical to understanding dental implant surgery. The oral cavity is made up of multiple interrelated components, including the teeth, gums, jawbone, and surrounding tissues. Each of these components is critical to the success of dental implants throughout time.

Dental, Gum, And Jawbone Structures

The teeth are made up of multiple layers: enamel, dentin, and pulp. The outermost layer, enamel, is the toughest component in the human body, protecting the below layers from injury.

The majority of the tooth structure is made up of dentin, which lies underneath the enamel. It supports and stabilizes the teeth. The pulp, which is found in the core of the tooth, includes nerves, blood vessels, and connective tissues.

The gums, also known as gingiva, surround the teeth and function as a barrier against germs and other potentially hazardous substances. Healthy gums are vital for tooth stability and dental implant support.

The jawbone, notably the alveolar bone, acts as the basis for the teeth and is essential in dental implant surgery. It offers essential support and stability during implant insertion. Additionally, the density and quality of the jawbone play an important role in determining the effectiveness of dental implants. Insufficient bone density or poor bone quality might result in implant failure or difficulties during surgery.

The Importance Of Bone Density And Quality

Bone density refers to the quantity of mineral content found in bone tissue. Higher bone density often suggests a stronger and more stable bone structure, which is required to support dental implants. Adequate bone density promotes good osseointegration, which is the process by which the implant fuses with the surrounding bone tissue, resulting in long-term stability and functioning.

Bone quality describes the overall health and integrity of bone tissue. Bone structure, architecture, and vascularity are all factors that influence bone quality. Healthy bone tissue facilitates effective implant placement while lowering the risk of problems like implant loosening or failure.

How Dental Anatomy Affects Implant Placement

The structure of the mouth cavity has a direct impact on the placement of dental implants. During the initial diagnostic and treatment planning phase, dentists consider a variety of anatomical parameters to identify the best position for implant implantation. Bone density, bone quality, tooth location, and occlusal connection are all considered to achieve optimal results.

When the jawbone lacks sufficient density or quality, bone grafting treatments may be required to supplement the bone tissue and provide enough support for implant implantation. Advanced imaging tools, including as cone beam computed tomography (CBCT), allow dentists to view the underlying anatomy and determine accurate implant placement procedures.

Understanding the complex link between oral anatomy and implant placement is critical for accomplishing successful dental implant surgery. By taking into account numerous anatomical parameters and using innovative procedures, dentists can assure the long-term success and stability of dental implants, restoring function and beauty to the patient's smile.

CHAPTER 3

Assessment And Planning For Implants

Initial Consultation And Assessment

Before undergoing dental implant surgery, you will normally have an initial consultation and examination with your dentist or oral surgeon. This step is critical since it establishes the framework for the whole treatment procedure. During this consultation, your dentist will take the time to learn about your dental requirements and preferences. They will inquire about your dental and medical history, including any current diseases or drugs you are using.

In addition to discussing your medical history, your dentist will thoroughly examine your dental health. They will examine your teeth, gums, and jawbone to decide if you are a good candidate for dental implants. This examination may include taking imprints of your teeth and mouth to develop models for future assessment.

Furthermore, your dentist will discuss your treatment objectives and expectations. They will discuss the advantages and dangers of dental implant surgery, as well as other treatment choices accessible to you. This open communication is critical to ensure that you are completely informed and comfortable with the planned treatment plan.

Diagnostic Tools Include X-Rays And CT Scans

To correctly assess your oral health and arrange for dental implant surgery, your dentist will use a variety of diagnostic technologies, including X-rays and CT scans. These imaging methods give extensive information about your jawbone's shape, neighboring tooth location, and general oral tissue health.

X-rays, such as panoramic or periapical radiographs, let your dentist determine the density and quality of your jawbone. This information is critical for establishing implant feasibility and detecting possible issues such as bone resorption or sinus involvement.

In addition to typical X-rays, your dentist may suggest a CT scan (computed tomography) for a more thorough examination. CT scans provide three-dimensional pictures of your oral anatomy, allowing for exact measurements and comprehensive views of bone structure. With this sophisticated imaging technology, your dentist can more accurately anticipate possible obstacles and arrange the ideal placement of dental implants.

Your dentist may create a specific treatment plan based on information from diagnostic equipment such as X-rays and CT scans.

Factors Influencing Treatment Planning

Several variables impact the treatment planning process for dental implant surgery, with bone health and medical history being among the most important.

Bone health is crucial to the success of dental implant therapy. A sufficient amount and density of bone are required to provide strong support for the implants and guarantee long-term stability and performance. If there are bone inadequacies, your dentist may propose bone grafting operations to supplement the existing bone and provide a solid foundation for implant implantation.

Your medical history is very important to consider while considering treatments. Certain medical diseases, like as diabetes or autoimmune disorders, might disrupt the healing process and raise the risk of complications after dental implant surgery. Similarly, drugs such as bisphosphonates and immunosuppressants might affect bone metabolism and hence therapy results.

During the assessment, your dentist will carefully analyze these aspects and how they affect your treatment plan. They may work with other healthcare experts, including your primary care physician or specialists, to ensure that your medical requirements are adequately handled throughout the implant placement procedure.

A Collaborative Approach Between Dentists And Surgeons

Successful dental implant surgery requires a joint effort between your dentist and oral surgeon. While your dentist is in charge of the initial examination, treatment planning, and restoration stages, an oral surgeon is normally responsible for the surgical placement of the implants.

This collaborative connection guarantees that all aspects of your therapy are carefully planned and maximized for success. Your dentist and oral surgeon will collaborate to explain treatment objectives, exchange diagnostic information, and schedule treatments.

Throughout the therapy process, open communication amongst all individuals involved is critical for addressing issues and altering the treatment plan as necessary. Working as a team, your dentist and oral surgeon can offer you thorough care and achieve the best results for your dental implant surgery.

CHAPTER 4

Types Of Dental Implants

Difference Between Endosteal And Subperiosteal Implants

Dental implants are available in a variety of varieties, each providing a distinct function depending on the individual's demands. Endosteal and subperiosteal implants are two of the basic classes, with considerable differences in location and attachment to the jawbone.

Endosteal Implants are the most prevalent form of dental implant. They are surgically implanted directly in the jawbone. These titanium implants serve as prosthetic tooth roots, giving a solid basis for replacement teeth. Endosteal implants are appropriate for most individuals who have adequate jawbone density.

To safely place the implant, the process entails drilling into the jawbone. Once the implant has healed and fused with the bone, a prosthetic tooth or dental crown is affixed to it.

Subperiosteal Implants: Unlike endosteal implants, which are embedded in the jawbone, subperiosteal implants are put on top of the jawbone, just behind the gum tissue. This kind of implant is advised for individuals who do not have enough bone height or density to sustain conventional implants. Subperiosteal implants are made of a metal framework that lies on the jawbone, with posts protruding through the gums to keep the prosthetic teeth in place. In certain situations, this method removes the requirement for bone grafting, making it an attractive choice for patients suffering from bone loss.

Materials For Implant Construction

The materials used in dental implant creation have a significant impact on their performance, longevity, and compatibility with the body. The most frequent materials are titanium and ceramic.

Titanium is the chosen material for dental implants because of its biocompatibility, strength, and ability to join with surrounding bone tissue via a process known as osseointegration. This metal is very robust and corrosion-resistant, making it ideal for long-term usage in the oral cavity. Titanium implants have been extensively investigated and shown to have success rates in dental implant surgery.

Ceramic implants are becoming more popular as an alternative to titanium implants, particularly among patients with metal sensitivity or cosmetic concerns. Ceramic implants, which are made from biocompatible materials like zirconia, provide natural-looking results while also being resistant to plaque accumulation and discoloration. While ceramic implants may not integrate as well with the bone as titanium implants, they remain a viable alternative for many individuals seeking dental repair.

Implant Shapes And Sizes

Dental implants are available in a variety of forms and sizes to meet individuals' varying demands and the unique architecture of their mouths. The form and size of the implant are determined by criteria such as the lost tooth's location, accessible bone, and desired cosmetic result.

Dental implants come in a variety of forms, including screw, cylinder, and blade designs. Screw-shaped implants are the most popular and adaptable, providing stability and simplicity of insertion in a variety of jawbone forms. Cylindrical implants are often utilized in narrow ridges or locations of restricted space.

Blade-shaped implants, on the other hand, are ideal for replacing numerous teeth in a row or supporting dentures.

Sizes: Implants are available in various sizes to match the proportions of the original teeth they replace. The diameter and length of the implant are critical factors during the treatment planning stage. Smaller implants may be utilized in regions with limited space or bone volume, while bigger implants provide more stability and support for chewing forces. The dentist will examine the patient's oral architecture and bone structure to select the proper implant size for the best outcomes.

Choosing The Correct Type Of Implant For Specific Cases

The patient and the dental care team work together to choose the best kind of dental implant for their needs, taking into consideration criteria such as the patient's oral health, bone density, medical history, and treatment objectives.

Case-Specific Considerations: Every patient has unique circumstances that must be carefully considered while selecting the appropriate kind of implant. The position and number of missing teeth, the quality of the surrounding gums and bone, and any previous dental work or prosthesis will all play a role in the choosing process.

Consultation and examination: Before dental implant surgery, patients have a thorough examination that includes dental exams, X-rays, and sometimes CT scans to check bone density and anatomical features. During the consultation, the dentist will go over treatment choices with the patient, such as the best kind of implant for their requirements, possible risks and advantages, and projected results.

Customized Treatment Plans: Based on the assessment results and the patient's choices, the dental team creates a personalized treatment plan that includes the implant insertion technique, the kind of restoration (crown, bridge, or denture), and the timetable for treatment. Collaboration between the patient and dental specialists guarantees that the selected implant satisfies the patient's functional and cosmetic needs while also fostering long-term oral health and happiness.

CHAPTER 5

Preparing For Surgery

Preoperative Instructions And Guidelines

Before having dental implant surgery, be sure to follow the pre-operative instructions supplied by your dentist or oral surgeon. These recommendations are intended to ensure the procedure's success while minimizing the danger of problems.

One of the key pre-operative instructions is to fast for 8 to 12 hours before the procedure. This helps to avoid anesthesia-related problems and lowers the risk of aspiration during the treatment. Your dentist may also recommend that you avoid certain drugs or supplements that might increase the risk of bleeding or interfere with the anesthetic.

It is important to notify your dentist about any current medical issues or drugs you are taking since they might impair the operation and healing process. Your dentist may need to modify your treatment plan or talk with your doctor to guarantee your safety throughout the operation.

Importance Of Oral Hygiene Before Surgery

Maintaining proper oral hygiene before dental implant surgery is critical for assuring the procedure's success and reducing the risk of infections. Your dentist will most likely prescribe thorough brushing and flossing to eliminate plaque and germs from your teeth and gums.

In addition to good oral hygiene, your dentist may recommend an antibacterial mouthwash to take before surgery. This helps to minimize the bacterial load in your mouth, lowering the risk of post-operative infections.

If you have any pre-existing dental disorders, such as gum disease or cavities, your dentist may advise you to treat them before undergoing implant surgery. Treating these concerns in advance may improve the general health of your mouth and increase the success rate of the implants.

Potential Lifestyle Adjustments

Making some lifestyle changes before dental implant surgery might help with a smoother recovery and better results. One key change is to change your diet to include soft meals that are simple to chew and will not put undue strain on the surgical site.

Your dentist may also advise you to stop smoking before surgery since it might hinder recovery and raise the chance of problems. Nicotine reduces blood flow to the gums and bone, which might disrupt the osseointegration process (the union of the implant with the jawbone).

In addition to diet and smoking cessation, it is critical to arrange for appropriate rest after surgery. Avoiding intense activity and having enough of rest may aid in healing and alleviate pain throughout the recovery process.

Anesthesia Options And Their Implications

Dental implant surgery may be conducted under local anesthetic, sedation, or general anesthesia, depending on the procedure's complexity and the patient's preferences. Each anesthetic choice has repercussions and concerns.

Local anesthesia is the process of numbing the surgical site using an anesthetic injection. It permits you to be awake throughout the process while preventing you from feeling any discomfort. This method is routinely utilized for simple implant placements and is linked with low risks and adverse effects.

Sedation anesthesia is the process of providing medicines to help you relax and feel sleepy during surgery. While you may stay aware, you will most likely have little or no recall of the surgery later. Sedation anesthesia is appropriate for people who have dental anxiety or are having more complex implant operations.

General anesthesia creates unconsciousness, leaving you fully oblivious and unresponsive throughout the operation. It is usually reserved for complicated situations or people who cannot tolerate local anesthetic or sedation. General anesthesia has a greater risk of complications and requires close monitoring by an anesthesiologist.

Before choosing an anesthetic, your dentist will consider your medical history, the difficulty of the procedure, and your degree of anxiety or comfort. They will go over the ramifications of each choice and help you make an educated selection based on your specific requirements and preferences.

CHAPTER 6

Surgical Procedure

Step-By-Step Explanation Of Implant Implantation

Implant implantation is a laborious process that includes several critical phases to ensure the procedure's success.

1. Initial Examination and Assessment: Before surgery, your dentist will do a complete examination of your mouth, including X-rays and perhaps CT scans, to determine the bone density and structure of the jaw.

2. Planning: Based on the findings of the evaluation, your dentist will develop a thorough treatment plan that specifies the exact position for implant placement. This design considers the size and form of the implant, as well as any existing dental concerns.

3. Anesthesia: Before the procedure, a local anesthetic will be delivered to numb the region where the implant will be put. In certain situations, sedation may be administered to help you relax throughout the process.

4. Incision: After numbing the region, your dentist will make a tiny incision in the gum tissue to reveal the bone below. This provides greater access to the implant location.

5. Drilling: Using sophisticated dental drills, your dentist will make a precise hole in the jawbone to put the implant. The hole depth and angle will be carefully determined to guarantee the implant's stability and alignment.

6. Implant Placement: The dental implant, which looks like a little screw, is gently put into the hole in the jawbone. To achieve a tight fit, gently tap or apply pressure.

7. Closing the Incision: After the implant is in place, the gum tissue is stitched together around it. These sutures facilitate healthy healing and avoid infection.

8. Healing phase: Following surgery, a healing phase is required to enable the implant to merge with the surrounding bone. This procedure, known as osseointegration, usually takes a few months.

9. Final Restoration: Once the implant has completely merged with the bone, a dental crown, bridge, or denture may be connected to it to restore oral function and aesthetics.

Surgical Techniques

Flapless surgery

Flapless surgery is a less invasive procedure that does not need gum tissue incisions. Using a sophisticated surgical guide, the implant is put straight through the gum tissue rather than raising a flap to expose the bone.

Because there are no sutures to remove, this method minimizes post-operative pain and accelerates recovery.

Guided Surgery

Guided surgery uses modern technology, such as 3D imaging and computer-guided surgical templates, to accurately arrange the placement of dental implants. Your dentist may use guided surgery to correctly establish the best location, angle, and depth for each implant before the procedure starts. This not only improves the procedure's accuracy but also lowers the danger of complications and provides predictable results.

Bone Grafting, Sinus Augmentation

If the jawbone is not robust or thick enough to support dental implants, bone grafting or sinus augmentation may be required.

Bone Grafting: This procedure includes transferring bone from another region of the body or utilizing synthetic bone material to enhance the existing jawbone. This creates a firm foundation for the implant to be put in and promotes long-lasting stability.

Sinus Augmentation: If the sinuses are too near to the upper jawbone, a sinus augmentation may be done to raise the sinus floor and provide more room for implant implantation. This surgery often includes inserting bone graft material into the sinus cavity to improve its height and volume.

Suturing And Closing The Surgical Site

Sutures are used to seal the surgical incision after the implant has been implanted and any required bone grafting or sinus augmentation has been accomplished.

Suturing Techniques: Your dentist will employ a variety of suturing methods to guarantee adequate wound closure and promote optimum healing. These might include procedures like interrupted sutures, which are individually tied knots, or continuous sutures, which use a single, continuous length of suture material. The procedure used is determined by the size and location of the incision, as well as the dentist's preferences.

Post-operative Care: Following surgery, it is critical to follow your dentist's post-operative care guidelines, which include taking any recommended medicines, avoiding certain foods, and keeping the surgical area clean. This minimizes pain, lowers the chance of complications, and promotes effective recovery.

CHAPTER 7

Postoperative Care And Recovery

Immediate Post-Operative Instructions

Following dental implant surgery, it is critical to follow quick post-operative recommendations to guarantee optimal healing and reduce problems. Your dentist or oral surgeon will offer particular advice adapted to your situation, however, you should anticipate the following basic instructions:

1. **Bleeding:** It is typical to have some bleeding after surgery. To stop the bleeding, gently bite down on the gauze supplied by the dentist. Replace the gauze as required until the bleeding has subsided. Avoid aggressive rinsing or spitting, since this might exacerbate bleeding.

2. Pain Management: You may feel discomfort or pain after surgery. Your dentist will most likely prescribe pain medication to relieve any discomfort. Take the drug exactly as advised, and avoid taking aspirin since it might cause bleeding.

3. Swelling: Swelling around the surgical site is normal and often occurs within 48 hours after surgery. To minimize swelling, apply an ice pack to the afflicted region for 20 minutes on and 20 minutes off during the first 24 hours. After 24 hours, use moist heat to assist relieve pain.

4. Rest and Recovery: Rest is required for good recovery. Avoid intense activity in the days after surgery, and keep your head elevated while resting down to avoid swelling.

5. Oral Hygiene: Keep your mouth clean, but be careful around the surgery site to prevent compromising the healing process.

Use a soft-bristled toothbrush and rinse with a moderate saltwater solution or your dentist's recommended mouthwash.

6. Dietary Restrictions: For the first several days following surgery, eat a soft or watery diet to prevent placing pressure on the surgical site. Avoid hot, spicy, or harsh meals that may irritate the skin.

7. Avoid Smoking and drinking: Smoking and drinking may disrupt the healing process and increase the likelihood of problems. It is advised to avoid smoking and drinking throughout the healing time.

Following these quick post-operative guidelines may help promote healthy healing and reduce pain after dental implant surgery.

Managing Pain And Discomfort

Pain and discomfort are typical after dental implant surgery, but there are various ways you may employ to successfully manage these symptoms.

1. Take Pain Medication: Your dentist will most likely prescribe pain relievers to help you feel better. Even if you are not in severe pain, take the medicine exactly as prescribed to avoid future agony.

2. Apply Ice Packs: Applying ice packs to the afflicted region helps decrease swelling and numb it, offering pain relief. Wrap the ice pack in a towel and place it on the outside of your face for 20 minutes on and 20 minutes off for the first 24 hours following surgery.

3. Use Over-the-counter Pain Relievers: In addition to any prescription pain medication, you may take over-the-counter pain relievers like ibuprofen or acetaminophen to aid with discomfort. Follow the dosage directions on the package carefully.

4. Rest: Rest is essential for the healing process, so take it easy and avoid intense activity during the first few days after surgery. To minimize swelling, try to elevate your head while resting down.

5. Follow Post-Operative Instructions: Following your dentist's post-operative instructions, which include food restrictions and oral hygiene habits, may assist in reducing pain and promote normal healing.

If you are experiencing severe or prolonged pain after dental implant surgery, see your dentist or oral surgeon for additional examination and treatment.

Diet Recommendations During The Healing Phase

Proper diet is critical to the healing process after dental implant surgery. Here are some food suggestions during the recovery phase:

1. Stick to Soft Foods: To prevent placing pressure on the surgical site in the days after surgery, eat soft or watery foods. Choose soups, yogurt, mashed potatoes, scrambled eggs, and smoothies.

2. Avoid Hard or Crunchy Foods: These foods might irritate the surgery site and slow recovery. Avoid nuts, chips, raw vegetables, and tough meats until your dentist has cleared you to resume a normal diet.

3. Drink lots of fluids, such as water and herbal teas, to remain hydrated throughout the healing process. Avoid drinks that are excessively hot or too cold, since they might irritate the surgical site.

4. Limit Sugar Consumption: Sugary meals and drinks might raise the risk of infection and slow recovery. Reduce your consumption of sugary snacks and beverages and replace them with healthy options.

5. Follow Your Dentist's Recommendations: Your dentist may give you particular dietary instructions depending on your unique requirements and the scope of your operation. Follow these guidelines carefully to encourage normal recovery and reduce problems.

You may help the healing process and improve the outcome of your dental implant surgery by adhering to these dietary guidelines.

Follow-Up Appointments And Tracking Progress

Following dental implant surgery, you must schedule follow-up consultations with your dentist or oral surgeon to check your progress and guarantee adequate healing. Here's what to anticipate during these appointments:

1. **Post-Operative Evaluation:** At your follow-up consultations, your dentist will inspect the surgical site to evaluate healing progress and look for indicators of problems including infection or implant failure.

2. **X-rays:** Your dentist may use X-rays to assess the location of the dental implants and guarantee good integration with the surrounding bone.

3. Adjustments: If required, your dentist may modify your treatment plan depending on your healing process. This might include changing your dental hygiene practice, dietary advice, or pain management techniques.

4. Long-Term Care Planning: Your dentist will talk with you about how to care for and maintain your dental implants in the long run, including appropriate oral hygiene, frequent dental check-ups, and possible future procedures.

5. Addressing Concerns: If you have any concerns or questions concerning your recuperation or dental implants, please share them with your dentist during follow-up sessions. They are there to help you through the recovery process.

Attending follow-up sessions and constantly monitoring your progress can guarantee the success of your dental implant surgery, allowing you to enjoy the advantages of a healthy, functioning smile for years.

CHAPTER 8

Potential Complications And How To Manage Them

Common Complications

Implant surgery, like other medical procedures, has hazards. The most prevalent consequences are infection and implant failure. Infection may arise during or after surgery if correct sterilizing standards are not followed or if the patient does not practice excellent oral hygiene thereafter. Implant failure may occur for several causes, including low bone quality, inappropriate implant placement, or inability to integrate with the jawbone.

Symptoms of infection include swelling, redness, discomfort, and, in rare cases, fever. If you suffer any of these symptoms, consult your dentist or oral surgeon right away.

Early treatment may prevent the infection from spreading and creating further difficulties.

Implant failure might appear as loosening of the implant, chronic pain or discomfort, or trouble chewing. In certain situations, the implant may have to be removed and replaced. Your dentist will evaluate the problem and suggest the best course of action to resolve the implant failure.

Early Signs Of Complications And When To Seek Help

Recognizing early indicators of problems is critical for proper management. If you have any of the following symptoms after implant surgery, please consult your dentist or oral surgeon:

1. Prolonged Pain: While some discomfort is expected after surgery, prolonged or worsening pain may suggest a problem.

2. **Swelling:** Swelling near the implant site might indicate infection or inflammation.

3. **Bleeding:** Excessive bleeding or bleeding that does not cease within a few hours should be treated immediately.

4. **Difficulty Chewing or Speaking:** If you are having problems chewing or speaking regularly after the first healing phase, there might be a problem with the implant.

5. **Loose Implant:** If you observe any movement or instability in the implant, this may suggest implant failure.

If you encounter any of these symptoms, please visit your dentist or oral surgeon. They can assess your situation and recommend the best line of action to resolve the issue.

Strategies To Minimize Risks During And After Surgery

While difficulties may arise, some techniques may assist limit the risks associated with implant surgery:

1. Choose a Qualified Provider: Look for a dentist or oral surgeon who has expertise with implant placement and a track record of success.

2. Follow Pre- and Post-Operative recommendations: Following your dentist's recommendations before and after surgery will assist improve healing and minimize the risk of problems.

3. Maintain Good Oral Hygiene: Proper oral hygiene is essential for avoiding infection and aiding healing after surgery. Brush and floss regularly, and follow the directions for any prescription mouthwashes or oral rinses.

4. Avoid Smoking and Alcohol: Smoking and drinking excessively may hinder healing and raise the risk of complications. It is advised to avoid these drugs, particularly during the first recovery phase.

5. Attend Follow-Up visits: Schedule regular follow-up visits with your dentist so that they can monitor your progress and handle any difficulties that occur as soon as possible.

By using these measures, you may reduce the risk of problems and increase the chances of a satisfactory result after implant surgery.

Long-Term Management Of Complications

Complications might emerge months or even years following implant surgery. Long-term treatment of problems often requires a collaborative approach from the patient and their dental care team.

For example, if an implant fails due to bone loss or poor bone quality, further treatments, such as bone grafting, may be required to provide appropriate support. Your dentist or oral surgeon will evaluate your specific circumstances and offer the best treatment option.

Regular dental check-ups are necessary to maintain the health of your implants and detect any possible issues early on. Your dentist will do a comprehensive examination and may propose diagnostic testing such as X-rays or CT scans to determine the integrity of the implants and surrounding structures.

Although difficulties may arise after implant surgery, early detection, and timely action can help reduce their effect and increase the probability of a good result. Follow your dentist's recommendations, practice proper oral hygiene, and attend frequent follow-up visits to help guarantee the long-term success of your dental implants.

CHAPTER 9

Dental Implant Maintenance And Long-Term Care

Importance Of Dental Hygiene For Implant Longevity

Maintaining proper oral hygiene is critical to the long-term success of dental implants. Implants, like natural teeth, may acquire plaque and bacteria if not properly maintained. This accumulation may cause gum disease and other issues, jeopardizing the implant's durability.

To prolong the life of your implants, maintain a strict dental hygiene practice. This involves cleaning your teeth at least twice per day with a soft-bristled toothbrush and fluoride toothpaste. Pay particular attention to the region around the implant, and clean it properly to minimize plaque formation.

Flossing is essential for implant maintenance. Use dental floss or interdental brushes to clean between the implants and adjacent teeth, removing any food particles and debris that your toothbrush may have missed. This helps to avoid the spread of gum disease and inflammation surrounding the implant.

In addition to everyday oral hygiene, regular dental check-ups are necessary to maintain the condition of your implants. Your dentist will examine the implant, surrounding gums, and bone structure to verify that everything is in excellent condition. They may also suggest professional cleanings to remove any hardened plaque (tartar) that cannot be eliminated with regular brushing and flossing.

By emphasizing oral cleanliness and scheduling periodic dental checkups, you may dramatically extend the life of your dental implants and retain a healthy, attractive smile for many years.

Regular Check-Ups And Professional Cleaning

Regular check-ups and expert cleanings are essential parts of dental implant care. These sessions enable your dentist to check on the health of your implants, identify any problems early on, and give the required treatments to guarantee their long-term success.

During a normal check-up, your dentist will carefully inspect your implants, gums, and jawbone to look for symptoms of inflammation, infection, or bone loss. They may also use X-rays to evaluate the bone density and integrity around the implant.

Professional cleaning is also essential for implant upkeep. Despite your best efforts with at-home oral hygiene, certain places may remain tough to reach and clean efficiently. Dental hygienists employ specialized equipment to remove plaque and tartar from the implant and the gumline, lowering the risk of gum disease and peri-implantitis.

In addition to cleaning, your dental hygienist may provide individualized oral hygiene instructions and ideas for improving your at-home care regimen. This may include suggestions for oral care items or practices that are suited to your requirements.

By scheduling frequent check-ups and expert cleanings, you can proactively treat any difficulties that may occur with your dental implants, ensuring they stay healthy and functioning for years.

Addressing Issues Such As Peri-Implantitis

Peri-implantitis is a dangerous illness that may threaten the success of dental implants if not managed. It is characterized by inflammation and infection of the tissues around the implant, which may result in bone loss and implant failure.

Early identification and treatments are critical for controlling peri-implantitis and avoiding future problems. If you suffer symptoms like redness, swelling, discomfort, or bleeding surrounding the implant, you should seek immediate dental treatment.

Your dentist will do a comprehensive examination to identify the severity of the irritation and the best course of therapy. Nonsurgical therapies that eradicate germs and aid healing may include professional cleanings, antimicrobial therapy, or laser therapy.

In more severe situations, surgery may be required to address bone loss and restore implant site health. This might include operations like bone grafting or implant surface cleaning to encourage new bone development and stabilize the implant.

In addition to receiving expert treatment, keeping good oral hygiene is critical for controlling peri-implantitis and avoiding recurrence. Your dentist may prescribe certain oral hygiene products or procedures to help maintain the implant site clean and bacteria-free.

By treating peri-implantitis early and according to your dentist's treatment and maintenance instructions, you may ensure the long-term success of your dental implants while also maintaining your oral health.

Tips To Protect Implants From Damage

While dental implants are intended to be strong and long-lasting, they are nonetheless susceptible to injury if not properly cared for. To safeguard your implants and optimize their longevity, consider the following suggestions:

1. Avoid chewing on hard items: Biting down on hard objects like ice, pencils, or fingernails might exert too much pressure on the implants, possibly damaging them.

2. Wear a mouthguard: If you engage in activities that may cause face damage, such as contact sports, a mouthguard may help protect your implants and natural teeth from harm.

3. Quit smoking: Smoking has been related to a higher risk of implant failure and comorbidities such as peri-implantitis. Quitting smoking may help your implants last longer and improve your overall dental health.

4. Maintain a consistent oral hygiene program, including daily brushing and flossing, to keep your implants clean and free of plaque and germs.

5. Schedule regular dental appointments for expert cleanings and inspections to monitor the health of your implants and handle any concerns as they arise.

By following these guidelines and taking proactive steps to safeguard your implants, you may help guarantee that they stay strong, stable, and functioning for many years.

CHAPTER 10

Future Advancements In Dental Implant Technology

Current Trends And Research In Implant Dentistry

Implant dentistry is a continuously growing subject, with academics and practitioners working to improve procedures and results. One of the current developments in implant dentistry is the development of less invasive treatments. These techniques are designed to lessen patient pain and recovery time while delivering efficient tooth replacement options.

Another development is the use of computer-aided implant surgery. This technology enables dentists to accurately arrange the placement of dental implants with modern imaging methods.

Dentists may increase the stability and endurance of implants by precisely mapping the patient's anatomy ahead of time.

Furthermore, research is concentrating on the development of innovative implant materials that enable quicker integration into the jawbone while lowering the risk of problems like infection or implant failure. These materials might include bioactive coatings or biomimetic surfaces that imitate the features of dental enamel and bone.

Additionally, there is significant interest in using stem cells and tissue engineering approaches to improve implant success rates. Researchers want to speed up the healing process and increase the long-term durability of dental implants by tapping into the body's inherent regenerative capabilities.

Overall, current developments and research in implant dentistry are targeted at improving treatment efficiency, predictability, and patient satisfaction.

By remaining up to date on these breakthroughs, dentists may provide their patients with the most modern and effective treatment choices available.

Predicted Advancements In Materials And Techniques

The future of dental implant technology seems optimistic, with advances in both materials and methods. One area of research is the creation of biocompatible materials that closely resemble the natural characteristics of teeth and bone. These materials might be improved ceramics, polymers, or composites designed to integrate better with the surrounding tissues.

In terms of approaches, robotic-assisted implant surgery is set to transform the sector. Using robotic technology, dentists may achieve exceptional precision and accuracy in implant placement, resulting in better results and a lower risk of problems.

Furthermore, developments in imaging technology, like as cone beam computed tomography (CBCT) and intraoral scanners, will allow dentists to get very comprehensive 3D pictures of their patients' oral anatomy. This degree of accuracy will allow for improved treatment planning and more predictable results from dental implant surgeries.

Another projected improvement is the widespread use of additive manufacturing, or 3D printing, to create unique implant components. This technique enables the manufacture of patient-specific implants with complex geometries that would be hard to create using regular manufacturing processes.

Overall, the future of dental implant technology offers great opportunities to improve treatment results and patient satisfaction. By adopting these innovations, dentists may offer their patients safer, more effective, and aesthetically acceptable tooth replacement options.

The Potential Impact Of Technology

Technology has the potential to transform every element of dental implant surgery, from diagnostic and treatment planning to postoperative care. One of the most important benefits of technology is the ability to tailor therapy to each patient's specific anatomy and oral health demands.

For example, 3D printing technology enables the creation of personalized surgical guides and implant components based on the patient's anatomy. This degree of customization improves the precision and predictability of implant placement, resulting in superior long-term results.

Furthermore, advances in imaging technology, such as CBCT and virtual planning software, allow dentists to see their patients' oral anatomy in unprecedented depth. This not only increases treatment planning accuracy but also facilitates more effective communication among dental experts engaged in the patient's care.

Nanotechnology is another area of technological innovation that has the potential to drastically alter dental implant surgery. Researchers may build nanoscale materials to generate surfaces that encourage quicker integration with surrounding tissues and minimize the danger of bacterial colonization, resulting in higher implant success rates.

Overall, using technology in dental implant surgery has the potential to improve patient care, increase treatment results, and expedite the whole procedure. By adopting these developments, dentists can give their patients with the best treatment possible.

Implications For Patient Care And Treatment Outcomes

Advancements in dental implant technology have far-reaching ramifications for patient care and treatment results.

One of the most important advantages is the possibility of providing patients with more comfortable and convenient treatment alternatives.

For example, minimally invasive procedures and computer-guided surgery lessen surgical trauma and post-operative suffering, enabling patients to recuperate faster and return to regular activities sooner.

Furthermore, the use of sophisticated materials and processes increases the lifespan and success rates of dental implants, minimizing the need for expensive and time-consuming retreatment treatments in the future.

Furthermore, technology enables improved communication and coordination among members of the dental team, resulting in more coordinated and complete treatment for patients. This multidisciplinary approach guarantees that all elements of the patient's oral health are evaluated throughout the treatment planning process, resulting in more predictable results and increased patient satisfaction.

Overall, using technology in dental implant surgery has the potential to improve the patient experience by increasing treatment efficiency, comfort, and effectiveness. Dentists may give the best possible care to their patients and achieve optimum treatment results by remaining up to date-on these innovations.

Conclusion

Finally, both patients and practitioners must comprehend dental implant surgery. Throughout this thorough guide, we've looked at the delicate process of restoring smiles and improving oral health with dental implants.

First and foremost, dental implant surgery provides a dependable and long-term option for those experiencing tooth loss. Unlike typical dentures or bridges, implants offer a permanent basis for replacement teeth, matching the natural structure of the teeth while encouraging stability and functioning. This restoration of function not only improves chewing and speaking abilities but also increases confidence and self-esteem by restoring a natural-looking grin.

Furthermore, the success of dental implant surgery is strongly dependent on meticulous planning and execution.

To get the best outcomes, every step, from the first consultation to the final implant placement, must be thoroughly planned. Advanced imaging tools, like as CT scans and digital impressions, help with the planning phase, allowing for accurate implant placement and reducing the chance of problems.

Furthermore, good post-operative care is critical to the long-term success of dental implants. Patients must maintain rigorous oral hygiene habits and attend frequent follow-up consultations to track the healing process and identify any problems early on. Furthermore, lifestyle variables like smoking and poor diet may have a detrimental influence on implant integration and must be addressed to improve results.

Importantly, dental implant surgery has dangers and restrictions. Infection, implant failure, and nerve damage are all possible complications, emphasizing the significance of working with a qualified and experienced dental implant expert. Certain medical illnesses and lifestyle choices may also have an impact on implant surgical eligibility, necessitating the consideration of alternate treatment alternatives.

Dental implant surgery is a huge innovation in contemporary dentistry, providing a permanent remedy for tooth loss that restores both function and aesthetics. Patients who grasp the complexity of the implant procedure and adhere to correct pre-operative planning and post-operative care may achieve good results and enjoy the advantages of a healthy, attractive smile for years to come. However, it is critical to approach implant surgery with realistic expectations and collaborate carefully with a trained dental practitioner to develop the best treatment strategy for your specific circumstances.

THE END

www.ingramcontent.com/pod-product-compliance
Lightning Source LLC
Chambersburg PA
CBHW071837210526
45479CB00001B/180